THE HYPERTHYROIDISM DIET COOKBOOK: NATURAL REMEDIES AND RECIPES

Enjoy Relief from Autoimmune Disorders, Graves' Disease, Hashimoto's Thyroiditis and Other Related Illnesses

Audrey McAllister, MD

COPYRIGHT PAGE

Requests for permission to use or reproduce any part of this publication should be addressed to the publisher in writing. The publisher reserves the right to grant or deny permission at their discretion, taking into consideration factors such as the intended use, nature of the excerpt, and potential impact on the original work.

Unauthorized reproduction or distribution of copyrighted material is a violation of intellectual property rights and may result in legal consequences. Individuals or entities found to be in breach of copyright law may be subject to legal action, including but not limited to injunctions, damages, and legal fees.

It is the responsibility of all users of this publication to familiarize themselves with and abide by copyright laws and regulations. By accessing or using any part of this work, individuals agree to comply with the terms and conditions set forth by the publisher regarding copyright protection and usage rights.

Table of Contents

INTRODUCTION

Welcome to an enriching culinary expedition crafted specifically for individuals navigating the challenges of hyperthyroidism. This cookbook emerges from a heartfelt intention to extend a helping hand to those grappling with this condition, aiming to offer not just sustenance, but also a pathway to harmony and a renewed sense of well-being through mindful dietary choices.

Hyperthyroidism, also known as an overactive thyroid, occurs when the thyroid gland produces an excess of hormones, particularly triiodothyronine (T3) and thyroxine (T4), which are essential for regulating various bodily functions. This butterfly-shaped gland sits at the front of the neck and plays a crucial role in hormone production, influencing metabolism and overall health.

This condition, which affects approximately 1 out of 100 Americans aged 12 and older, can have widespread effects on the body, necessitating intervention from a healthcare professional. Symptoms of hyperthyroidism, such as weight loss, hand tremors, and irregular heartbeat, stem from the heightened metabolic rate caused by an excess of thyroid hormones.

The thyroid's role in regulating metabolism is pivotal, as it determines how cells utilize energy. When there's an overproduction of T3, T4, or both, it disrupts the body's equilibrium, leading to various discomforts. It's crucial to diagnose and address hyperthyroidism promptly to alleviate symptoms and prevent potential complications.

The prevalence of hyperthyroidism is higher in women, occurring about 10 times more frequently than in men, typically manifesting between the ages of 20 and 40. Despite its small size, the thyroid exerts significant influence over bodily functions, including heart rate and body temperature. Excessive hormone production can result in significant health issues that may require medical intervention.

SECTION 1: WHAT EXACTLY IS HYPERTHYROIDISM?

Hyperthyroidism, a condition marked by an overactive thyroid gland, stems from an imbalance in thyroid hormone production. Nestled like a delicate butterfly at the front of the neck, the thyroid gland wields significant influence over numerous bodily functions, including metabolism, energy regulation, heart rate, body temperature, and the smooth operation of various organs.

When this gland kicks into overdrive, churning out excessive quantities of thyroid hormones thyroxine (T4) and triiodothyronine (T3), the result is hyperthyroidism. These hormones, crucial for regulating metabolic rate and energy usage at the cellular level, now propel the body into a state of hyperactivity, setting off a cascade of symptoms and challenges.

Graves' disease, a common autoimmune disorder, often stands as the culprit behind hyperthyroidism, as it mistakenly attacks the thyroid gland, prompting it to go into overproduction mode. Other factors such as thyroid nodules, thyroid inflammation (thyroiditis), and certain medications can also contribute to this thyroid frenzy.

The symptoms of hyperthyroidism present in a myriad of ways, reflecting the broad impact of heightened thyroid hormone levels on the body. Weight loss despite increased appetite due to a revved-up metabolism, a racing heart accompanied by palpitations, excessive sweating even in cool environments, muscle weakness and fatigue despite increased metabolic activity—all telltale signs of this condition.

Mental health can also take a hit, with symptoms like heightened anxiety, restlessness, and difficulty concentrating often accompanying hyperthyroidism. Physical manifestations such as hand tremors and sleep disturbances further underscore the pervasive effects of this hormonal imbalance.

In women, menstrual cycles may undergo alterations, resulting in lighter or less frequent periods. Some individuals may even develop a visible enlargement of the thyroid gland, known as goiter.

In severe cases, hyperthyroidism can escalate into a thyroid storm, characterized by severe symptoms and potentially life-threatening consequences, including cardiac issues and osteoporosis due to rapid bone turnover.

Diagnosis typically involves blood tests to measure levels of thyroid hormones (T3, T4) and thyroid-stimulating hormone (TSH), a pituitary gland hormone that regulates thyroid function. Treatment options range from medication and radioactive iodine therapy to surgical removal of part or all of the thyroid gland, with ongoing medical monitoring and lifestyle adjustments forming key components of management.

Seeking prompt medical attention for diagnosis and treatment is crucial for individuals experiencing symptoms of hyperthyroidism. With appropriate medical support, many people can effectively manage their thyroid health and lead fulfilling lives despite this condition's challenges.

Origins and Factors of Risk

There's a wealth of understanding around some of the root causes of hyperthyroidism, but the deeper we delve, the more mysteries we uncover. At its core, this condition often stems from an excessive production of thyroxine (T4) and triiodothyronine (T3), both vital thyroid hormones, due to a disruption in their usual regulation. Accurate diagnosis, effective treatment, and preventative measures hinge on unraveling the intricacies of what triggers hyperthyroidism and the factors that elevate its risks.

One well-known culprit behind hyperthyroidism is Graves' disease, an autoimmune disorder where the body mistakenly directs its immune system to attack the thyroid gland. This relentless assault prompts the gland to go into overdrive, churning out excessive thyroid hormones and setting off hyperthyroidism. The familial clustering of Graves' disease suggests a genetic predisposition, but environmental factors and stressors may also conspire to trigger its onset.

Another pathway to hyperthyroidism can be paved by thyroid nodules, innocuous growths that take root within the thyroid gland. While most nodules are benign, some have a knack for autonomously producing hormones, leading to hyperactivity in the thyroid. Though usually harmless, the possibility of malignancy underscores the importance of comprehensive evaluation and diagnosis.

Inflammation can also tip the thyroid scales towards hyperthyroidism, as seen in cases of thyroiditis. This temporary hyperthyroid state arises when the thyroid gland becomes inflamed, releasing stored hormones into the bloodstream. Culprits for triggering thyroiditis can range from viral infections to hormonal fluctuations post-pregnancy, and even certain medications.

Additionally, an excessive intake of iodine can potentially push individuals already predisposed to hyperthyroidism over the edge. Since thyroid hormones rely on iodine for their synthesis and regulation, an excess of this mineral can throw off the delicate balance, fueling hyperthyroidism.

In the grand tapestry of hyperthyroidism, each thread we unravel reveals more complexity and nuance. Understanding the diverse array of triggers and risk factors is paramount not only for pinpointing the roots of this condition but also for devising tailored treatment plans and preventive strategies. By delving deeper into the labyrinth of hyperthyroidism, we inch closer to mastering its mysteries and offering holistic care to those affected by its grip.

Dangers on the Horizon

Hyperthyroidism tends to occur more frequently in women than in men, particularly among women of reproductive age. Furthermore, the risk of developing hyperthyroidism increases with age, with individuals over 60 being particularly susceptible to this condition. Additionally, the onset of hyperthyroidism, particularly Graves' disease, may be influenced by a family history of the condition. Those with a family history of autoimmune diseases such as type 1 diabetes or celiac disease are at an even higher risk.

Individuals with hyperthyroidism often experience Graves' disease and thyroid eye disease, both of which are commonly associated with this condition. Interestingly, research has shown a correlation between cigarette smoking and an increased risk of developing these conditions in individuals with hyperthyroidism. Moreover, hyperthyroidism can be triggered by various factors such as stress and certain illnesses, particularly in individuals who have a genetic predisposition to autoimmune disorders.

In some cases, pregnant women may develop temporary hyperthyroidism due to hormonal shifts during pregnancy. It's important to recognize that the causes and risk factors of hyperthyroidism can interact in complex ways. Therefore, obtaining a correct diagnosis and initiating appropriate treatment require a comprehensive medical evaluation.

This evaluation should include blood tests to assess thyroid hormone levels and thyroid-stimulating hormone (TSH) levels. Early identification and treatment of hyperthyroidism are crucial to prevent complications and maintain optimal thyroid function. If you suspect that you may have hyperthyroidism or are at risk due to your family history or other factors, it's essential to seek medical assistance promptly. By addressing hyperthyroidism proactively, individuals can effectively manage their condition and improve their overall health and well-being.

Hyperthyroidism Principles and Guidelines

Ensuring effective management of hyperthyroidism requires a multifaceted approach that integrates medical treatment with lifestyle adjustments and adherence to principles that promote thyroid health and overall well-being. By embracing these concepts and incorporating them into your daily routine, you can enhance your quality of life, support thyroid function, and gain better control over symptoms.

Seeking proper diagnosis and personalized therapy is paramount, and this typically involves consultation with a qualified medical specialist, often an endocrinologist. Treatment options may include antithyroid drugs, beta-blockers to regulate heart rate and palpitations, radioactive iodine therapy to reduce thyroid hormone production, or surgical removal of part or all of the thyroid gland. Regular visits to your healthcare provider are essential for monitoring thyroid health, adjusting treatment plans as needed, and addressing any concerns you may have.

In addition to medical intervention, maintaining a balanced diet is crucial for supporting thyroid function and overall health. Aim to consume a diverse array of foods, including whole grains, lean proteins, fruits, vegetables, and healthy fats. While minerals like iodine, selenium, and zinc are important for thyroid health, it's important to avoid excessive intake, as this can exacerbate hyperthyroidism. Limiting stimulants such as caffeine and nicotine can also help alleviate symptoms.

Your doctor may recommend a low-iodine diet in conjunction with radioactive iodine therapy to optimize treatment outcomes. This may involve avoiding iodized salt, shellfish, dairy products, and certain processed foods. If prescribed antithyroid medication, it's crucial to adhere to the prescribed dosage and schedule, as these drugs help normalize thyroid hormone levels and require ongoing monitoring.

Incorporating stress-reduction techniques like meditation, deep breathing, yoga, and mindfulness can complement medical treatment by alleviating symptoms and supporting overall well-being. Regular exercise is also beneficial for weight management, mental health, and cardiovascular function, although individuals with cardiac issues should consult their healthcare provider before starting an exercise regimen.

Be mindful of foods that may affect thyroid function, such as goitrogens found in cruciferous vegetables, soy products, and some fruits. While these foods can be consumed in moderation if cooked or lightly steamed, it's important to be aware of their potential impact on thyroid health. Regular monitoring of thyroid hormone levels, including TSH, T3, and T4, is essential to evaluate treatment efficacy and maintain thyroid function within a healthy range.

Hydration is key for symptom management and overall health, as adequate water intake can help alleviate fatigue and muscle weakness associated with hyperthyroidism. Educating yourself about hyperthyroidism and actively participating in your own care by asking questions and communicating openly with your healthcare provider can empower you to make informed decisions and optimize treatment outcomes.

Hyperthyroidism is a complex condition with varying treatment needs, and successful management requires individualized care tailored to your specific circumstances. By integrating these recommendations into your daily routine in collaboration with your healthcare team, you can support thyroid health, manage symptoms effectively, and improve your overall quality of life.

SECTION 2: HANDLING HYPERTHYROIDISM THROUGH DIET

When managing hyperthyroidism through diet, it's crucial to select foods that support thyroid health, alleviate symptoms, and promote overall well-being. While dietary adjustments can play a significant role in managing the condition and enhancing quality of life, they should complement rather than replace conventional medical treatment.

The thyroid gland relies on iodine for hormone synthesis, but excessive intake of this mineral can worsen hyperthyroidism symptoms. Striking a balance is key. Individuals with hyperthyroidism induced by Graves' disease should steer clear of iodine-rich foods like iodized salt, shellfish, and seaweed.

Furthermore, it's wise to moderate consumption of cruciferous vegetables such as broccoli, cabbage, and cauliflower, as well as soy products and millet, due to their goitrogenic properties, which can disrupt thyroid function. Cooking or gentle steaming can help neutralize these effects.

Prioritizing nutrient-dense foods like whole grains, lean meats, fruits, and vegetables is essential. These foods are packed with vitamins, minerals, and antioxidants that promote optimal health.

Selenium, an essential micronutrient for thyroid and immune function, can be found in foods like Brazil nuts, shellfish, eggs, and whole grains, and can help improve thyroid function.

Incorporating omega-3 fatty acid-rich foods such as fatty fish, flaxseeds, and walnuts into the diet can help manage inflammation associated with hyperthyroidism.

Avoiding caffeine and other stimulants is advisable, as they can exacerbate symptoms like palpitations and anxiety. Tailoring meals to include a balance of carbohydrates, proteins, and healthy fats can help stabilize blood sugar levels and provide sustained energy throughout the day.

Adequate hydration is crucial for overall health and can help alleviate symptoms like fatigue and muscle weakness.

Individuals experiencing rapid metabolism and weight loss may benefit from consuming smaller, more frequent meals throughout the day. Being mindful of hunger and fullness cues can facilitate better control over food intake and weight management.

Minimizing intake of sugary and highly processed foods can help stabilize blood sugar levels and reduce symptom severity.

Before making significant dietary changes, it's important to consult with a healthcare professional or registered dietitian specializing in thyroid health. They can offer personalized guidance based on individual health needs and circumstances.

It's essential to recognize that hyperthyroidism is a complex condition that requires individualized treatment. What works for one person may not work for another. Dietary modifications should be part of a comprehensive approach to managing the condition, alongside conventional medical care and a healthy lifestyle.

By being mindful of the impact of diet on hyperthyroidism and working closely with healthcare professionals, individuals can take control of their condition and improve their quality of life.

Eating Out with Hyperthyroidism: Navigating Healthy Choices

Ensuring your dining experience supports your thyroid health, especially when dealing with hyperthyroidism, involves a blend of mindfulness, preparation, and educated choices. Although eating out can pose challenges, it's entirely feasible to relish meals that cater to your dietary requirements and promote thyroid well-being.

Before stepping into a restaurant, take a moment to explore the menu online, if feasible. Seek out options that are less likely to be high in iodine (if advised) or contain goitrogenic properties. Familiarize yourself with healthier selections such as lean proteins, vegetables, whole grains, and minimally processed items.

Restaurants are often willing to accommodate special dietary needs. Don't hesitate to request modifications to suit your preferences. For example, ask for steamed veggies instead of fried sides, request sauces on the side, or substitute iodine-rich ingredients.

Opt for lean protein sources like grilled chicken, fish, or tofu. These choices offer essential amino acids without excessive fat or iodine content.

Be cautious of high-sodium foods, which can exacerbate hyperthyroidism symptoms. Request dishes with reduced salt, or ask the chef to prepare your meal with less salt.

When available, choose whole grain options such as brown rice or whole wheat bread. These alternatives provide fiber and sustained energy without causing rapid blood sugar spikes.

Portions at restaurants tend to be larger than those typically consumed at home. Consider sharing a dish with a friend or asking for a to-go box when your meal arrives, setting aside a portion for later.

Strive to include a variety of vegetables in your meal to obtain essential nutrients, fiber, and antioxidants vital for overall health.

Beware of hidden sources of iodine or goitrogens in dressings, sauces, or condiments. Requesting these items on the side enables you to manage your intake better.

Opt for hydrating choices like water, herbal tea, or unsweetened beverages, avoiding added sugars or stimulants.

Steer clear of high-sugar beverages, as they can disrupt blood sugar levels and worsen symptoms. Choose drinks without added sugars and limit caffeine intake.

Listen to your body's signals. If a dish doesn't align with your dietary needs, explore other menu options or consider dining elsewhere.

Practice mindful eating by savoring each bite, eating slowly, and paying attention to how different foods affect you.

Consider having a balanced snack before heading to the restaurant to prevent overindulging on less healthy options.

Inform your dining companions about your dietary preferences or restrictions to ensure a more comfortable experience and foster understanding.

Approach dining out with intention, making thoughtful choices that support your thyroid health goals. Remember, your well-being takes precedence, and making informed decisions contributes to your overall health and quality of life.

Foods to Embrace and Evade

Types of Foods to Eat

Ensuring optimal thyroid function and alleviating symptoms of hyperthyroidism can be supported by incorporating specific foods into your diet. By prioritizing nutrient-rich options abundant in vitamins, minerals, and antioxidants, you can provide your body with the necessary tools to maintain a healthy balance.

Whole grains, such as quinoa, brown rice, and whole wheat, serve as excellent sources of sustained energy and essential dietary fiber, aiding in digestion and overall well-being. Lean proteins like poultry, fish, lentils, and tofu contribute vital amino acids crucial for sustaining optimal health and supporting bodily functions.

Diversifying your plate with a vibrant array of fruits and vegetables offers a spectrum of vitamins and minerals essential for bolstering the immune system and fostering a well-rounded diet. Embracing a colorful assortment ensures you're receiving a wide range of nutrients necessary for maintaining overall health.

Incorporating selenium-rich foods like Brazil nuts, shellfish, and eggs into your meals can further enhance thyroid function, as selenium plays a pivotal role in regulating thyroid hormones. Additionally, embracing omega-3 fatty acids from sources like flaxseeds and fatty fish such as salmon and mackerel can impart anti-inflammatory effects, supporting overall health and well-being.

Furthermore, prioritizing fermented foods like sauerkraut and Greek yogurt can contribute to gut health, fostering a balanced microbiome crucial for immune modulation and overall wellness. By nourishing your gut, you support a robust immune system and aid in the absorption of essential nutrients, promoting optimal health from within.

In essence, by making mindful choices and incorporating these nutrient-dense foods into your daily diet, you can proactively support thyroid health, alleviate symptoms of hyperthyroidism, and cultivate overall well-being. Remember, your diet serves as a powerful tool in nurturing your body and optimizing your health for the long term.

Limit or avoid these foods

Numerous food items have been associated with exacerbating symptoms of hyperthyroidism and potentially disrupting thyroid function. To mitigate these effects, it's advisable to moderate the intake of iodine-rich foods such as seaweed, shellfish, and iodized salt. Similarly, cruciferous vegetables like broccoli, cabbage, and cauliflower, along with soy products, which have the potential to induce goiter, should be consumed in moderation or briefly boiled.

Moreover, substances like caffeine and other stimulants can exacerbate feelings of nervousness and heart palpitations. Considering this, it might be beneficial to limit or altogether avoid the consumption of stimulants such as coffee, soda, energy drinks, and certain prescription medications. Additionally, reducing the consumption of processed foods and sugary meals can contribute to maintaining stable blood sugar levels, thereby promoting overall health.

It's important to acknowledge that hyperthyroidism presents differently in each individual, and what works well for one person may not be suitable for another. Hence, tailoring one's diet to individual requirements and symptoms is crucial. Seeking guidance from a healthcare professional or a qualified dietitian specializing in thyroid health can facilitate this process. By actively participating in managing one's condition and prioritizing balanced, nutritious meals that support thyroid function, individuals can take proactive steps toward maintaining their overall well-being.

Maintaining Thyroid Health Through Nutrient Balance

Ensuring the optimal function of your thyroid gland demands careful attention to your dietary choices, particularly when navigating conditions such as hyperthyroidism. The production of thyroid hormones and the regulation of metabolism hinge on specific nutrients that should take center stage in your diet, not only to support your thyroid but also to bolster your overall well-being.

One crucial component for thyroid health is iodine, a fundamental ingredient for thyroid hormone synthesis. While iodine is indispensable for proper thyroid function, excessive intake can exacerbate symptoms of hyperthyroidism. It's crucial to strike a balance. Incorporate iodine-rich foods like iodized salt, shellfish, and dairy into your diet in moderate amounts. However, if your hyperthyroidism stems from Graves' disease, consulting with your healthcare provider about your iodine intake is advisable.

Selenium plays a pivotal role in converting the inactive thyroid hormone (T4) into its active form (T3), thereby promoting thyroid health. Foods rich in selenium, such as Brazil nuts, seafood, eggs, and whole grains, can support thyroid function. However, ensuring you get the right amount of selenium can be challenging.

Zinc also contributes to thyroid hormone synthesis and function. While zinc is present in nuts, seeds, whole grains, lean meats, and poultry, maintaining a balanced diet is essential for supporting both your thyroid and immune system.

Inflammation associated with hyperthyroidism can be managed with anti-inflammatory omega-3 fatty acids.

Including fatty fish like salmon, flaxseeds, chia seeds, walnuts, and olive oil in your diet can help maintain a healthy thyroid and reduce inflammation.

Vitamins A and D play vital roles in supporting both the immune system and thyroid health. Incorporating foods rich in vitamin A, such as sweet potatoes, carrots, and dark leafy greens, as well as sources of vitamin D like sunlight, fatty fish, and fortified foods, can be beneficial.

Antioxidants found in fruits and vegetables combat oxidative stress and promote immune system and thyroid health. Therefore, incorporating a variety of antioxidant-rich fruits and vegetables into your diet is essential.

A well-rounded diet that includes a balance of carbohydrates, proteins, and healthy fats is crucial for maintaining overall health, blood sugar regulation, and sustained energy levels.

Staying adequately hydrated is also vital for optimal thyroid function and overall well-being. Ensuring you consume enough water throughout the day can help your body function more efficiently.

It's important to recognize that individual nutritional needs vary, and consulting with a healthcare professional or registered dietitian specializing in thyroid health can help determine the optimal dietary balance for your specific situation. By focusing on these key nutrients and maintaining open communication with your healthcare provider, you can support optimal thyroid function and enhance your quality of life.

SECTION 3: SPECIAL CONSIDERATIONS FOR HYPERTHYROIDISM

Successfully managing hyperthyroidism and improving overall health requires careful consideration and attention to various factors that encompass not only dietary choices but also lifestyle habits and overall well-being. By addressing these aspects, individuals can enhance their ability to control hyperthyroidism and promote thyroid health effectively.

One significant factor to consider is the impact of stress on hyperthyroidism symptoms. Incorporating relaxation practices such as meditation, deep breathing exercises, yoga, and mindfulness techniques can not only alleviate stress but also contribute to promoting thyroid health. Prioritizing rest and finding moments of enjoyment in daily life can also have positive effects on both physical and mental well-being.

Regular physical activity is another key component of managing hyperthyroidism and supporting overall health. Engaging in exercise offers numerous benefits, including weight management, cardiovascular health improvement, and enhancement of mental well-being. However, individuals with underlying cardiac issues should approach high-intensity workouts with caution and consult with their healthcare provider before initiating or modifying their fitness routine.

The importance of quality sleep cannot be overstated when it comes to thyroid health. Establishing a consistent sleep schedule, creating a relaxing sleep environment, and practicing relaxation techniques can help ensure adequate restorative sleep, which is crucial for maintaining thyroid function.

Hyperthyroidism can also affect heart health, leading to irregular heartbeats or palpitations. It is essential to seek evaluation and treatment from a qualified medical professional for heart-related symptoms. Limiting consumption of stimulants such as caffeine and maintaining moderation in their intake can help manage heart-related symptoms associated with hyperthyroidism.

For individuals prescribed antithyroid medication, adherence to the prescribed regimen is critical for regulating thyroid hormone levels effectively. Regular monitoring of thyroid function through tests such as TSH, T3, and T4 levels is necessary to evaluate the efficacy of treatment and adjust medication as needed. Any adverse reactions or concerns should be promptly communicated to a healthcare provider.

Lifestyle factors such as smoking and excessive alcohol consumption can adversely affect thyroid health and should be avoided. Educating oneself about hyperthyroidism, treatment options, and associated risks empowers individuals to take an active role in managing their condition. Seeking support from friends, family, or support groups can provide invaluable emotional and moral support during the challenges of managing hyperthyroidism.

It's important to recognize that hyperthyroidism manifests differently in each individual, and treatment approaches may vary accordingly. Collaborating with a healthcare provider to tailor a treatment plan that considers individual circumstances, symptoms, and preferences is essential for effectively managing hyperthyroidism while prioritizing overall health and well-being. By addressing these unique factors, individuals can optimize their health outcomes and effectively manage hyperthyroidism.

Metabolism and Weight Management

Navigating weight management with hyperthyroidism presents unique challenges due to the heightened metabolic rate and energy expenditure often associated with the condition. For individuals grappling with these challenges, achieving and maintaining a healthy weight requires a multifaceted approach that encompasses medical guidance, dietary adjustments, and lifestyle modifications.

First and foremost, establishing a close partnership with your healthcare provider is essential when addressing weight fluctuations linked to hyperthyroidism. Your healthcare team can conduct thorough evaluations, including assessing thyroid hormone levels and overall health, to tailor a comprehensive treatment plan that addresses both your metabolism and symptom relief.

Embracing a balanced and nutritious diet is a cornerstone of managing hyperthyroidism and weight control. Opting for whole, unprocessed foods rich in lean proteins, complex carbohydrates, healthy fats, vitamins, and minerals is paramount. Paying attention to portion sizes ensures that your body receives adequate nourishment without disrupting metabolic balance.

Additionally, adopting a strategy of more frequent meals can help stabilize blood sugar levels and prevent excessive energy expenditure. This approach is particularly beneficial for individuals experiencing rapid weight loss and heightened metabolic rates.

Surprisingly, ensuring adequate calorie intake is crucial in managing hyperthyroidism-related weight loss. The increased energy demands of hyperthyroidism necessitate sufficient caloric intake to prevent muscle wasting and maintain overall health.

Prioritizing nutrient-dense foods packed with vitamins, minerals, and antioxidants supports overall well-being and helps regulate appetite, facilitating weight management. Incorporating lean protein sources like poultry, fish, lentils, and tofu into your diet aids in preserving muscle mass amidst heightened metabolic activity.

Hydration is another critical aspect of maintaining metabolic function and supporting weight management. Consistently consuming an adequate amount of water throughout the day helps sustain hydration levels and curbs unnecessary hunger.

Regular physical activity plays a pivotal role in weight management and overall health, although it's important to consult with your healthcare provider, especially if you experience heart-related symptoms.

Engaging in stress-reduction practices such as meditation, deep breathing, and mindfulness can also contribute to both weight stability and overall well-being.

Throughout your journey with hyperthyroidism, close collaboration with your healthcare team is paramount. Tailored advice and support based on your specific condition, symptoms, and treatment plan can guide you towards effective weight and metabolism management.

Practicing patience, self-compassion, and mindfulness is crucial in navigating the challenges of hyperthyroidism-related weight fluctuations. By prioritizing conscious food choices, stress management techniques, and regular communication with your healthcare team, you can empower yourself to achieve and maintain a healthy weight amidst the complexities of hyperthyroidism.

Remember, everyone's experience with hyperthyroidism is unique, but with a holistic approach centered on medical guidance, mindful lifestyle choices, and whole-person wellness, effective weight and metabolism management is achievable.

Navigating Food Sensitivities and Allergies

When navigating the complexities of hyperthyroidism, addressing dietary sensitivities and allergies becomes a crucial aspect requiring thoughtful consideration and a personalized approach. It's not uncommon for individuals with hyperthyroidism to encounter food sensitivities or allergies, given the condition's impact on the immune system and gut microbiota.

Hyperthyroidism can trigger fluctuations in the immune system, rendering individuals more susceptible to developing sensitivities or allergies. If you suspect that you may be experiencing such reactions, seeking guidance from a healthcare professional is paramount. Together, you can explore potential food triggers and devise strategies to manage them effectively.

The role of thyroid hormones extends beyond regulating metabolism; they also influence gut motility and digestion. Consequently, hyperthyroidism can influence gut health, potentially exacerbating issues related to food sensitivities and allergies. However, adopting a holistic approach to gut health through a well-rounded diet, probiotic supplementation (under medical supervision), and stress management can provide significant support.

In cases where a food allergy is suspected, an elimination diet may be recommended under the supervision of a healthcare provider. This involves temporarily removing potential allergens from the diet and gradually reintroducing them to identify triggers. It's essential to approach elimination diets with caution and expert guidance to ensure safety and efficacy.

For individuals with hyperthyroidism and concurrent dietary sensitivities or allergies, consulting with a dietitian experienced in managing thyroid conditions and restrictive diets is invaluable. A tailored diet plan can be crafted to meet nutritional needs while accommodating dietary restrictions, promoting both health and satisfaction.

Given the interplay between hyperthyroidism and immune system function, maintaining a diet rich in vitamins, minerals, and antioxidants is beneficial for supporting overall health and bolstering immune function. Emphasizing whole foods such as vegetables, fruits, lean proteins, and whole grains can contribute to immune resilience.

Collaboration with healthcare professionals, including primary care physicians and dietitians, is essential for individuals managing hyperthyroidism alongside dietary sensitivities or allergies. These experts can offer guidance on dietary modifications, ensure adequate nutrient intake, and monitor medication interactions and reactions.

For those dealing with food allergies, practicing meticulous kitchen hygiene and exercising caution when dining out are essential precautions to prevent allergic reactions. Thoroughly disinfecting surfaces and utensils can help minimize cross-contamination and reduce the risk of allergen exposure.

Developing mindfulness around eating habits can empower individuals to better understand how different foods impact their bodies. Keeping a food diary and noting any symptoms or changes following meals can provide valuable insights into individual dietary triggers and reactions.

It's important to recognize that responses to dietary allergies and sensitivities vary from person to person. What works for one individual may not be effective for another. Therefore, collaborative engagement with healthcare providers is crucial in developing a personalized approach to managing food sensitivities or allergies while effectively addressing hyperthyroidism and overall health.

SECTION 4: DOCTOR-APPROVED HYPERTHYROIDISM DIET RECIPES

BREAKFAST RECIPES FOR HYPERTHYROIDISM

Omelette with spinach and mushroom

What You Need

2 eggs

1 cup baby spinach

1/4 cup sliced mushrooms

1 tbsp. olive oil

Salt and pepper to taste

Directions

Whisk eggs in a small bowl and season with salt and pepper.

Heat olive oil in a non-stick pan over medium heat.

Add spinach and mushrooms to the pan and cook until the spinach is wilted and the mushrooms are tender.

Pour the egg mixture into the pan and cook until the bottom is set, then flip and cook until the other side is set.

Serve hot.

Greek yogurt with berries and chia seeds

What You Need

1 cup plain Greek yogurt

1/2 cup mixed berries (blueberries, raspberries, strawberries)

1 tbsp. chia seeds

Honey or maple syrup (optional)

Directions

Mix the Greek yogurt and chia seeds together in a bowl.

Top with mixed berries and drizzle with honey or maple syrup if desired.

Serve chilled.

Avocado toast with smoked salmon

What You Need

1 slice whole grain bread

1/4 avocado, mashed

1 oz. smoked salmon

1 tbsp. capers

Salt and pepper to taste

Directions

Toast the bread until golden brown.

Mash the avocado with a fork and spread it over the toast.

Top with smoked salmon and capers.

Season with salt and pepper to taste.

Serve immediately.

Scrambled eggs with tomato and basil

What You Need

2 eggs

1/2 cup chopped tomato

1 tbsp. chopped fresh basil

1 tbsp. butter

Salt and pepper to taste

Directions

Crack the eggs into a bowl and whisk until well beaten.

Heat butter in a non-stick pan over medium heat.

Add chopped tomato to the pan and cook until softened.

Pour the egg mixture into the pan and stir gently with a spatula until the eggs are scrambled and cooked through.

Stir in the chopped basil and season with salt and pepper to taste.

Serve hot.

Quinoa porridge with almond milk and cinnamon

What You Need

1/2 cup cooked quinoa

1/2 cup almond milk

1 tbsp. honey

1/4 tsp. ground cinnamon

Chopped nuts or dried fruit for topping (optional)

Directions

Combine cooked quinoa, almond milk, honey, and cinnamon in a small pot.

Cook over medium heat, stirring occasionally, until heated through and thickened to a porridge consistency.

Top with chopped nuts or dried fruit if desired.

Serve hot.

Buckwheat pancakes with almond butter and banana

What You Need

1/2 cup buckwheat flour

1/2 tsp. baking powder

1/4 tsp. salt

1/2 cup almond milk

1 egg

1 tbsp. maple syrup

1/2 banana, sliced

1 tbsp. almond butter

Directions

In a bowl, whisk together buckwheat flour, baking powder, and salt.

In another bowl, whisk together almond milk, egg, and maple syrup.

Add the wet ingredients to the dry ingredients and stir until well combined.

Heat a non-stick pan over medium heat.

Pour 1/4 cup of the batter onto the pan and cook until bubbles form on the surface, then flip and cook until the other side is golden brown.

Repeat with remaining batter.

Serve the pancakes topped with sliced banana and almond butter.

Turkey bacon with sautéed kale and sweet potato

What You Need

2 slices turkey bacon

1 cup chopped kale

1 small sweet potato, peeled and diced

1 tbsp. olive oil

Salt and pepper to taste

Directions

Cook the turkey bacon according to package instructions and set aside.

In a non-stick pan, heat olive oil over medium heat.

Add the chopped kale and diced sweet potato to the pan and cook until the kale is wilted and the sweet potato is tender.

Season with salt and pepper to taste.

Serve hot with the cooked turkey bacon.

Coconut milk smoothie with mango and ginger

What You Need

1/2 cup coconut milk

1/2 cup frozen mango chunks

1/2 banana

1/2-inch piece fresh ginger, peeled and grated

1 tbsp. honey

Directions

Combine all What You Need in a blender and blend until smooth.

Add more coconut milk or water if needed to achieve desired consistency.

Serve chilled.

Sardines on whole grain toast with sliced tomato

What You Need

2 slices whole grain bread

1 can sardines in oil, drained

1/2 tomato, sliced

Salt and pepper to taste

Directions

Toast the bread until golden brown.

Top each slice with sardines and sliced tomato.

Season with salt and pepper to taste.

Serve immediately.

Steamed broccoli and egg whites with brown rice

What You Need

1 cup cooked brown rice

1 cup broccoli florets

2 egg whites

1 tbsp. olive oil

Salt and pepper to taste

Directions

In a small pot, steam the broccoli florets until tender.

In a non-stick pan, heat olive oil over medium heat.

Add the egg whites to the pan and scramble until cooked through.

Season with salt and pepper to taste.

Serve the steamed broccoli and scrambled egg whites over the cooked brown rice.

Grilled chicken with roasted asparagus and sweet potato

What You Need

4 oz. boneless, skinless chicken breast

1 cup asparagus spears, trimmed

1 small sweet potato, peeled and diced

1 tbsp. olive oil

Salt and pepper to taste

Directions

Preheat a grill or grill pan to medium-high heat.

Season the chicken breast with salt and pepper and grill until cooked through, about 6-8 minutes per side.

Toss the asparagus and sweet potato with olive oil and season with salt and pepper.

Roast in the oven at 400°F for 15-20 minutes, or until tender.

Serve the grilled chicken with the roasted asparagus and sweet potato.

Almond flour muffins with blueberries and flaxseed

What You Need

1 cup almond flour

1/4 cup ground flaxseed

1/4 cup honey

1/4 cup unsweetened applesauce

2 eggs

1 tsp. baking powder

1/2 tsp. vanilla extract

1/2 cup fresh or frozen blueberries

Directions

Preheat the oven to 350°F and line a muff in tin with muffin liners.

In a mixing bowl, whisk together the almond flour, ground flaxseed, and baking powder.

In a separate bowl, beat the eggs and mix in the honey, applesauce, and vanilla extract.

Add the wet ingredients to the dry What You Need and stir until well combined.

Fold in the blueberries.

Pour the batter into the muffin cups, filling each about 3/4 full.

Bake for 20-25 minutes, or until a toothpick inserted into the center of a muffin comes out clean.

Allow to cool for a few minutes before serving.

Tuna salad with avocado and cucumber on whole grain crackers

What You Need

1 can tuna, drained

1/2 avocado, mashed

1/2 cucumber, diced

1 tbsp. chopped fresh parsley

Salt and pepper to taste

Whole grain crackers

Directions

In a mixing bowl, combine the drained tuna, mashed avocado, diced cucumber, and chopped parsley.

Season with salt and pepper to taste.

Serve the tuna salad with whole grain crackers on the side.

Spinach and feta omelette with sliced tomatoes

What You Need

2 eggs

1/2 cup fresh spinach, chopped

1 oz. crumbled feta cheese

1/2 tomato, sliced

Salt and pepper to taste

1 tsp. olive oil

Directions

In a small bowl, beat the eggs and season with salt and pepper.

Heat the olive oil in a non-stick pan over medium heat.

Add the chopped spinach to the pan and cook until wilted.

Pour the beaten eggs into the pan and cook until set, about 2-3 minutes.

Sprinkle the crumbled feta cheese over one half of the omelette.

Use a spatula to fold the omelette in half over the cheese.

Serve the omelette with sliced tomatoes on the side.

Chia seed pudding with raspberries and almonds

What You Need

1/4 cup chia seeds

1 cup unsweetened almond milk

1 tbsp. honey

1/4 cup fresh raspberries

1 tbsp. sliced almonds

Directions

In a mixing bowl, whisk together the chia seeds, almond milk, and honey.

Cover the bowl and refrigerate for at least 2 hours, or overnight.

Serve the chia seed pudding topped with fresh raspberries and sliced almonds.

Green smoothie with spinach and banana

What You Need

1 cup fresh spinach

1/2 banana

1/2 cup unsweetened almond milk

1/2 cup plain Greek yogurt

1 tbsp. honey

Directions

Combine all ingredients in a blender and blend until smooth.

Add more almond milk if needed to achieve desired consistency.

Serve chilled.

Brown rice cake with almond butter and sliced banana

What You Need

1 brown rice cake

1 tbsp. almond butter

1/2 banana, sliced

Directions

Spread the almond butter on top of the rice cake.

Top with sliced banana.

Serve immediately.

LUNCH RECIPES FOR HYPERTHYROIDISM

Grilled chicken salad with mixed greens, cucumbers, and cherry tomatoes

What You Need

4 oz grilled chicken breast

2 cups mixed greens

1/2 cucumber, sliced

1/2 cup cherry tomatoes, halved

2 tbsp balsamic vinaigrette

Directions

Season the chicken breast with salt and pepper, and grill until fully cooked.

Arrange the mixed greens on a plate and top with sliced cucumbers and halved cherry tomatoes.

Slice the grilled chicken breast and add to the salad.

Drizzle with balsamic vinaigrette and serve.

Baked salmon with steamed broccoli and brown rice

What You Need

4 oz salmon fillet

1 cup steamed broccoli

1/2 cup cooked brown rice

Salt and pepper to taste

Lemon wedges for serving

Directions

Preheat the oven to 375°F.

Season the salmon fillet with salt and pepper.

Place the salmon fillet on a baking sheet lined with parchment paper and bake for 12-15 minutes, or until fully cooked.

While the salmon is cooking, steam the broccoli.

Serve the salmon with steamed broccoli and cooked brown rice.

Squeeze fresh lemon juice over the salmon before serving.

Turkey and vegetable stir-fry with quinoa

What You Need

4 oz ground turkey

1 cup mixed vegetables (such as bell peppers, onions, and mushrooms)

1/2 cup cooked quinoa

1 tbsp olive oil

Salt and pepper to taste

Directions

Heat the olive oil in a large skillet over medium-high heat.

Add the ground turkey to the skillet and cook until browned, breaking it up with a spatula.

Add the mixed vegetables to the skillet and cook for 5-7 minutes, until they are tender.

Season with salt and pepper to taste.

Serve the turkey and vegetable stir-fry over cooked quinoa.

Grilled vegetables with whole grain pita bread and hummus

What You Need

2 cups mixed vegetables (such as zucchini, eggplant, bell peppers, and onions)

2 whole grain pita breads

1/2 cup hummus

1 tbsp olive oil

Salt and pepper to taste

Directions

Preheat a grill or grill pan over medium-high heat.

Toss the mixed vegetables with

1 tbsp of olive oil, salt, and pepper.

Grill the vegetables for 5-7 minutes, until they are tender and charred in spots.

Warm the pita breads on the grill for 1-2 minutes per side.

Serve the grilled vegetables with warm pita breads and hummus on the side.

Roasted turkey breast with roasted sweet potatoes and green beans

What You Need

4 oz roasted turkey breast

1 cup roasted sweet potatoes

1 cup roasted green beans

1 tbsp olive oil

Salt and pepper to taste

Directions

Preheat the oven to 400°F.

Season the turkey breast with salt and pepper and roast for 25-30 minutes, or until fully cooked.

While the turkey is roasting, toss the sweet potatoes and green beans with olive oil, salt, and pepper.

Roast the sweet potatoes and green beans on a baking sheet lined with parchment paper for 20-25 minutes, until they are tender and slightly browned.

Serve the roasted turkey breast with roasted sweet potatoes and green beans.

Tuna salad with mixed greens and a side of brown rice

What You Need

4 oz canned tuna, drained

2 cups mixed greens

1/2 cup cooked brown rice

1/4 cup chopped celery

1/4 cup chopped red onion

2 tbsp olive oil

1 tbsp lemon juice

Salt and pepper to taste

Directions

In a large bowl, combine the drained tuna, chopped celery, chopped red onion, olive oil, lemon juice, salt, and pepper.

Toss to combine.

Serve the tuna salad over a bed of mixed greens and a side of cooked brown rice.

Grilled chicken with roasted vegetables and quinoa

What You Need

4 oz grilled chicken breast

2 cups roasted vegetables (such as zucchini, bell peppers, and onions)

1/2 cup cooked quinoa

1 tbsp olive oil

Salt and pepper to taste

Directions

Season the chicken breast with salt and pepper and grill until fully cooked.

While the chicken is grilling, toss the mixed vegetables with olive oil, salt, and pepper.

Roast the mixed vegetables on a baking sheet lined with parchment paper for 15-20 minutes, until they are tender and slightly charred.

Serve the grilled chicken with roasted vegetables and cooked quinoa.

Black bean soup with a side salad of mixed greens and cucumbers

What You Need

1 can (15 oz) black beans, drained and rinsed

2 cups low-sodium chicken or vegetable broth

1 onion, chopped

2 cloves garlic, minced

1 tbsp olive oil

Salt and pepper to taste

2 cups mixed greens

1/2 cucumber, sliced

2 tbsp balsamic vinaigrette

Directions

Heat the olive oil in a large pot over medium-high heat.

Add the chopped onion and minced garlic to the pot and sauté until the onion is translucent.

Add the black beans and broth to the pot and bring to a boil.

Reduce the heat and simmer for 10-15 minutes, until the beans are tender.

Season with salt and pepper to taste.

Serve the black bean soup with a side salad of mixed greens and sliced cucumber dressed with balsamic vinaigrette.

Baked sweet potato with black beans and salsa

What You Need

1 medium sweet potato

1/2 cup canned black beans, drained and rinsed

1/4 cup salsa

1 tbsp olive oil

Salt and pepper to taste

Directions

Preheat the oven to 400°F.

Pierce the sweet potato several times with a fork and place it on a baking sheet lined with parchment paper.

Bake the sweet potato for 45-50 minutes, until it is tender and easily pierced with a fork.

While the sweet potato is baking, heat the black beans in a small saucepan over medium heat until warmed through.

Serve the baked sweet potato topped with black beans, salsa, and a drizzle of olive oil.

Chickpea and vegetable stir-fry with brown rice

What You Need

1 can (15 oz) chickpeas, drained and rinsed

2 cups mixed vegetables (such as broccoli, carrots, and bell peppers)

1 cup cooked brown rice

2 tbsp soy sauce

1 tbsp olive oil

Salt and pepper to taste

Directions

Heat the olive oil in a large skillet over medium-high heat.

Add the mixed vegetables to the skillet and stir-fry for 5-7 minutes, until they are tender-crisp.

Add the chickpeas to the skillet and stir-fry for an additional 2-3 minutes, until they are warmed through.

Season with soy sauce, salt, and pepper to taste.

Serve the chickpea and vegetable stir-fry over a bed of cooked brown rice.

Grilled salmon with roasted asparagus and a side of quinoa

What You Need

4 oz grilled salmon fillet

1 cup roasted asparagus

1/2 cup cooked quinoa

1 tbsp olive oil

Salt and pepper to taste

Directions

Season the salmon fillet with salt and pepper and grill until fully cooked.

While the salmon is grilling, toss the asparagus with olive oil, salt, and pepper.

Roast the asparagus on a baking sheet lined with parchment paper for 10-15 minutes, until they are tender and slightly browned.

Serve the grilled salmon with roasted asparagus and cooked quinoa.

Grilled shrimp with roasted vegetables and quinoa

What You Need

4 oz grilled shrimp

2 cups roasted vegetables (such as eggplant, zucchini, and bell peppers)

1/2 cup cooked quinoa

1 tbsp olive oil

Salt and pepper to taste

Directions

Season the shrimp with salt and pepper and grill until fully cooked.

While the shrimp is grilling, toss the vegetables with olive oil, salt, and pepper.

Roast the vegetables on a baking sheet lined with parchment paper for 10-15 minutes, until they are tender and slightly browned.

Serve the grilled shrimp with roasted vegetables and cooked quinoa.

Tuna salad with avocado and cucumber slices

What You Need

1 can (5 oz) tuna, drained

1 avocado, peeled and diced

1/2 cucumber, sliced

1 tbsp olive oil

Salt and pepper to taste

Directions

In a small bowl, combine the drained tuna with diced avocado and olive oil.

Season with salt and pepper to taste.

Serve the tuna salad with cucumber slices on the side.

Turkey and hummus wrap with baby carrots on the side

What You Need

3 oz sliced turkey breast

2 tbsp hummus

1 whole wheat wrap

1/2 cup baby carrots

Salt and pepper to taste

Directions

Lay the whole wheat wrap flat on a plate.

Spread hummus evenly over the wrap.

Arrange the sliced turkey on top of the hummus.

Season with salt and pepper to taste.

Roll up the wrap tightly and slice in half.

Serve the turkey and hummus wrap with baby carrots on the side.

Tofu stir-fry with brown rice and steamed broccoli

What You Need

4 oz firm tofu, cubed

2 cups broccoli florets

1 cup cooked brown rice

1 tbsp soy sauce

1 tbsp olive oil

Salt and pepper to taste

Directions

Heat the olive oil in a large skillet over medium-high heat.

Add the cubed tofu to the skillet and stir-fry for 5-7 minutes, until it is lightly browned on all sides.

Add the broccoli florets to the skillet and stir-fry for an additional 2-3 minutes, until they are tender-crisp.

Season with soy sauce, salt, and pepper to taste.

Serve the tofu and broccoli stir-fry over a bed of cooked brown rice.

Chicken and vegetable soup with a side of whole wheat crackers

What You Need

1 cup shredded cooked chicken breast

2 cups low-sodium chicken or vegetable broth

1 onion, chopped

2 cloves garlic, minced

2 cups mixed vegetables (such as carrots, celery, and green beans)

Salt and pepper to taste

Whole wheat crackers

Directions

In a large pot, combine the shredded chicken, chopped onion, minced garlic, mixed vegetables, and broth.

Bring the soup to a boil and reduce the heat to a simmer.

Simmer for 10-15 minutes, until the vegetables are tender.

Season with salt and pepper to taste.

Serve the chicken and vegetable soup with whole wheat crackers on the side.

DINNER RECIPES FOR HYPERTHYROIDISM

Grilled chicken with roasted vegetables

What You Need

4 chicken breasts

2 cups of mixed vegetables (e.g., carrots, zucchini, bell peppers)

1 tablespoon of olive oil

Salt and pepper to taste

Directions

Preheat oven to 375°F.

Season chicken breasts with salt and pepper.

Heat olive oil in a skillet over medium-high heat.

Cook chicken breasts for 6-8 minutes on each side or until cooked through.

While chicken is cooking, toss vegetables with olive oil, salt, and pepper.

Place vegetables on a baking sheet and roast for 20-25 minutes or until tender.

Serve chicken with roasted vegetables.

Baked salmon with quinoa and steamed broccoli

What You Need:

4 salmon fillets

1 cup of quinoa

2 cups of water

4 cups of broccoli florets

1 tablespoon of olive oil

Salt and pepper to taste

Directions

Preheat oven to 375°F.

Season salmon fillets with salt and pepper.

Place salmon fillets on a baking sheet and bake for 10-12 minutes or until cooked through.

Rinse quinoa and combine with water in a medium saucepan.

Bring to a boil, reduce heat to low, and simmer for 15-20 minutes or until quinoa is tender and water is absorbed.

Steam broccoli for 5-7 minutes or until tender.

Toss broccoli with olive oil, salt, and pepper.

Serve salmon with quinoa and steamed broccoli.

Stir-fried tofu and mixed vegetables with brown rice

What You Need:

1 block of tofu

2 cups of mixed vegetables (e.g., broccoli, bell peppers, mushrooms)

1 tablespoon of vegetable oil

1 tablespoon of soy sauce

1 tablespoon of cornstarch

Salt and pepper to taste

2 cups of cooked brown rice

Directions

Press tofu to remove excess moisture.

Cut tofu into cubes.

Toss tofu with cornstarch, salt, and pepper.

Heat vegetable oil in a wok or large skillet over high heat.

Add tofu and cook until crispy and browned on all sides.

Remove tofu from skillet.

Add mixed vegetables to skillet and stir-fry for 3-5 minutes or until tender.

Add soy sauce to vegetables and stir to combine.

Serve tofu and vegetables over brown rice.

Lentil soup with a side salad

What You Need:

2 cups of dried lentils

6 cups of water or vegetable broth

1 onion, chopped

2 garlic cloves, minced

1 carrot, chopped

1 celery stalk, chopped

1 tablespoon of olive oil

1 teaspoon of cumin

Salt and pepper to taste

Mixed greens for salad

Directions

Rinse lentils and add to a large pot with water or broth.

Bring to a boil, reduce heat, and simmer for 30-40 minutes or until lentils are tender.

While lentils are cooking, heat olive oil in a skillet over medium-high heat.

Add onion, garlic, carrot, and celery to skillet and sauté for 5-7 minutes or until vegetables are tender.

Add vegetables to lentil pot.

Season with cumin, salt, and pepper.

Serve with mixed greens on the side.

Grilled shrimp with zucchini noodles

What You Need:

1 pound of raw shrimp

3-4 medium zucchinis

2 tablespoons of olive oil

2 garlic cloves, minced

Salt and pepper to taste

Directions

Preheat grill to medium-high heat.

Rinse and pat dry shrimp.

Toss shrimp with olive oil, minced garlic, salt, and pepper.

Grill shrimp for 2-3 minutes on each side or until pink and cooked through.

While shrimp is cooking, use a spiralizer to create zucchini noodles.

Heat olive oil in a skillet over medium-high heat.

Add zucchini noodles to skillet and sauté for 3-5 minutes or until tender.

Season with salt and pepper.

Serve grilled shrimp over zucchini noodles.

Baked sweet potato topped with black beans and salsa

What You Need:

4 medium sweet potatoes

1 can of black beans, rinsed and drained

1 cup of salsa

Salt and pepper to taste

Directions

Preheat oven to 400°F.

Pierce sweet potatoes with a fork several times.

Place sweet potatoes on a baking sheet and bake for 40-50 minutes or until tender.

While sweet potatoes are cooking, heat black beans in a saucepan over medium heat.

Season with salt and pepper.

Once sweet potatoes are done, cut them open and top with black beans and salsa.

Serve immediately.

Roasted turkey breast with roasted Brussels sprouts and sweet potato

What You Need:

1 pound of turkey breast

1 pound of Brussels sprouts

2 sweet potatoes

2 tablespoons of olive oil

Salt and pepper to taste

Directions

Preheat oven to 375°F.

Rinse and pat dry turkey breast.

Rub turkey breast with olive oil and season with salt and pepper.

Place turkey breast in a baking dish and roast for 60-90 minutes or until internal temperature reaches 165°F.

While turkey is cooking, rinse and trim Brussels sprouts.

Cut sweet potatoes into 1-inch cubes.

Toss Brussels sprouts and sweet potatoes with olive oil, salt, and pepper.

Place vegetables on a baking sheet and roast for 20-25 minutes or until tender.

Serve turkey breast with roasted Brussels sprouts and sweet potato.

Veggie stir-fry with brown rice and cashews

What You Need:

2 cups of mixed vegetables (e.g., broccoli, carrots, bell peppers)

1 tablespoon of vegetable oil

2 garlic cloves, minced

2 tablespoons of soy sauce

1 tablespoon of cornstarch

1/4 cup of cashews

Salt and pepper to taste

2 cups of cooked brown rice

Directions

Heat vegetable oil in a wok or large skillet over high heat.

Add mixed vegetables and minced garlic to skillet and stir-fry for 3-5 minutes or until tender.

In a small bowl, whisk together soy sauce and cornstarch.

Add soy sauce mixture to skillet and stir to combine.

Add cashews and stir-fry for an additional 1-2 minutes.

Season with salt and pepper.

Serve stir-fry over brown rice.

Grilled steak with roasted root vegetables

What You Need:

1 pound of steak (e.g., sirloin, ribeye)

2 cups of mixed root vegetables (e.g., carrots, parsnips, sweet potatoes)

2 tablespoons of olive oil

Salt and pepper to taste

Directions

Preheat grill to medium-high heat.

Rinse and pat dry steak.

Rub steak with olive oil and season with salt and pepper.

Grill steak for 4-6 minutes on each side or until cooked to desired doneness

While steak is cooking, rinse and chop mixed root vegetables into 1-inch cubes.

Toss vegetables with olive oil, salt, and pepper.

Place vegetables on a baking sheet and roast in the oven for 20-25 minutes or until tender.

Let steak rest for 5-10 minutes before slicing.

Serve sliced steak with roasted root vegetables.

Baked salmon with roasted asparagus and quinoa

What You Need:

4 salmon fillets

1 bunch of asparagus

1 cup of quinoa

2 cups of water

2 tablespoons of olive oil

Salt and pepper to taste

Directions

Preheat oven to 375°F.

Rinse and pat dry salmon fillets.

Rub salmon fillets with olive oil and season with salt and pepper.

Place salmon fillets in a baking dish and bake for 12-15 minutes or until cooked through.

While salmon is cooking, rinse and trim asparagus.

Toss asparagus with olive oil, salt, and pepper.

Place asparagus on a baking sheet and roast for 10-12 minutes or until tender.

Rinse quinoa and place in a saucepan with water.

Bring quinoa to a boil over high heat, then reduce heat to low and simmer for 15-20 minutes or until water is absorbed.

Fluff quinoa with a fork.

Serve baked salmon with roasted asparagus and quinoa.

Grilled chicken with sautéed spinach and brown rice

What You Need:

4 chicken breasts

1 pound of spinach

2 tablespoons of olive oil

2 garlic cloves, minced

Salt and pepper to taste

2 cups of cooked brown rice

Directions

Preheat grill to medium-high heat.

Rinse and pat dry chicken breasts.

Rub chicken breasts with olive oil and season with salt and pepper.

Grill chicken breasts for 5-7 minutes on each side or until cooked through.

While chicken is cooking, rinse spinach and remove stems.

Heat olive oil in a skillet over medium-high heat.

Add minced garlic to skillet and sauté for 1-2 minutes or until fragrant.

Add spinach to skillet and sauté for 3-5 minutes or until wilted.

Season with salt and pepper.

Serve grilled chicken with sautéed spinach and brown rice.

Lentil soup with mixed greens salad

What You Need:

2 cups of lentils

8 cups of water

1 onion, chopped

2 carrots, chopped

2 celery stalks, chopped

2 garlic cloves, minced

2 bay leaves

2 teaspoons of dried thyme

Salt and pepper to taste

4 cups of mixed greens

2 tablespoons of balsamic vinegar

2 tablespoons of olive oil

Directions

Rinse lentils and place in a large pot with water, chopped onion, chopped carrots, chopped celery, minced garlic, bay leaves, dried thyme, salt, and pepper.

Bring lentil mixture to a boil over high heat, then reduce heat to low and simmer for 40-50 minutes or until lentils are tender.

While lentil soup is cooking, rinse and dry mixed greens.

In a small bowl, whisk together balsamic vinegar and olive oil to create dressing.

Toss mixed greens with dressing.

Serve lentil soup with mixed greens salad.

Grilled shrimp skewers with roasted vegetables

What You Need:

1 pound of shrimp, peeled and deveined

1 zucchini, sliced

1 red bell pepper, chopped

1 yellow onion, chopped

1 tablespoon of olive oil

Salt and pepper to taste

Directions

Preheat grill to medium-high heat.

Rinse and pat dry shrimp.

Thread shrimp onto skewers, alternating with slices of zucchini and chopped red bell pepper.

Brush skewers with olive oil and season with salt and pepper.

Grill skewers for 3-4 minutes on each side or until shrimp are pink and cooked through.

While skewers are cooking, rinse and chop yellow onion.

Toss onion with olive oil, salt, and pepper.

Place onion on a baking sheet and roast for 10-12 minutes or until tender.

Serve grilled shrimp skewers with roasted vegetables.

Tuna salad with mixed greens and roasted sweet potato

What You Need:

2 cans of tuna, drained

1/4 cup of mayonnaise

1 tablespoon of dijon mustard

2 celery stalks, chopped

2 green onions, chopped

Salt and pepper to taste

4 cups of mixed greens

2 sweet potatoes, peeled and chopped

1 tablespoon of olive oil

Directions

In a medium bowl, mix together drained tuna, mayonnaise, dijon mustard, chopped celery, chopped green onions, salt, and pepper.

Rinse and dry mixed greens.

Divide mixed greens among 4 plates.

Peel and chop sweet potatoes into 1-inch cubes.

Toss sweet potatoes with olive oil, salt, and pepper.

Place sweet potatoes on a baking sheet and roast for 20-25 minutes or until tender.

Serve tuna salad with mixed greens and roasted sweet potato.

Baked chicken with roasted brussels sprouts and wild rice

What You Need:

4 chicken thighs

1 pound of brussels sprouts

2 tablespoons of olive oil

Salt and pepper to taste

2 cups of cooked wild rice

Directions

Preheat oven to 375°F.

Rinse and pat dry chicken thighs.

Rub chicken thighs with olive oil and season with salt and pepper.

Place chicken thighs in a baking dish and bake for 35-40 minutes or until cooked through.

While chicken is cooking, rinse and trim brussels sprouts.

Toss brussels sprouts with olive oil, salt, and pepper.

Place brussels sprouts on a baking sheet and roast for 20-25 minutes or until tender.

Rinse wild rice and place in a saucepan with water.

Bring wild rice to a boil over high heat, then reduce heat to low and simmer for 35-40 minutes or until water is absorbed.

Fluff wild rice with a fork.

Serve baked chicken with roasted brussels sprouts and wild rice.

Grilled shrimp and vegetable kebabs with quinoa

What You Need:

1 pound of shrimp, peeled and deveined

1 red onion, chopped

1 red bell pepper, chopped

1 yellow bell pepper, chopped

1 zucchini, sliced

2 tablespoons of olive oil

Salt and pepper to taste

1 cup of quinoa

2 cups of water

Directions

Preheat grill to medium-high heat.

Rinse and pat dry shrimp.

Thread shrimp and chopped vegetables onto skewers.

Brush skewers with olive oil and season with salt and pepper.

Grill skewers for 3-4 minutes on each side or until shrimp are pink and cooked through.

While skewers are cooking, rinse quinoa and place in a saucepan with water.

Bring quinoa to a boil over high heat, then reduce heat to low and simmer for 15-20 minutes or until water is absorbed.

Fluff quinoa with a fork.

Serve grilled shrimp and vegetable kebabs with quinoa.

Broiled salmon with roasted asparagus and sweet potato mash

What You Need:

4 salmon fillets

1 pound of asparagus

2 tablespoons of olive oil

Salt and pepper to taste

2 sweet potatoes, peeled and chopped

1/4 cup of almond milk

Directions

Preheat broiler.

Rinse and pat dry salmon fillets.

Rub salmon fillets with olive oil and season with salt and pepper.

Place salmon fillets on a baking sheet and broil for 8-10 minutes or until cooked through.

While salmon is cooking, rinse and trim asparagus.

Toss asparagus with olive oil, salt, and pepper.

Place asparagus on a baking sheet and roast for 10-12 minutes or until tender.

Peel and chop sweet potatoes into 1-inch cubes.

Place sweet potatoes in a saucepan with water.

Bring sweet potatoes to a boil over high heat, then reduce heat to low and simmer for 15-20 minutes or until tender.

Drain sweet potatoes and mash with almond milk until smooth.

Serve broiled salmon with roasted asparagus and sweet potato mash.

SOUP RECIPES FOR HYPERTHYROIDISM

Broccoli Cheddar Soup:

What You Need

1 tablespoon olive oil

1 onion, chopped

2 cloves garlic, minced

4 cups broccoli florets

4 cups vegetable broth

1 cup shredded reduced-fat cheddar cheese

1 cup low-fat milk

Salt and pepper to taste

Directions

Heat olive oil in a large pot over medium heat. Add onion and garlic. Sauté for 5 minutes until onion is translucent.

Add broccoli florets and vegetable broth. Bring to a boil.

Reduce heat and simmer for 15 minutes until broccoli is tender.

Use an immersion blender or transfer a portion of the soup to a blender and blend until smooth.

Return soup to the pot. Add shredded cheddar cheese and milk. Stir until cheese is melted and soup is heated through.

Adjust seasoning if needed. Serve hot.

Tomato Basil Soup:

What You Need

1 tablespoon olive oil

1 onion, chopped

2 cloves garlic, minced

2 cans diced tomatoes

4 cups vegetable broth

1/4 cup fresh basil leaves, chopped

1/2 teaspoon dried oregano

Salt and pepper to taste

Directions

Heat olive oil in a large pot over medium heat. Add onion and garlic. Sauté for 5 minutes until onion is translucent.

Add diced tomatoes (with juice), vegetable broth, fresh basil, dried oregano, salt, and pepper. Bring to a boil.

Reduce heat and simmer for 20 minutes.

Use an immersion blender or transfer a portion of the soup to a blender and blend until smooth.

Adjust seasoning if needed. Serve hot.

Mushroom Barley Soup:

What You Need

1 tablespoon olive oil

1 onion, chopped

2 cloves garlic, minced

8 ounces mushrooms, sliced

1 carrot, diced

1 celery stalk, diced

1/2 cup pearl barley

4 cups vegetable broth

1 teaspoon dried thyme

Salt and pepper to taste

Directions

Heat olive oil in a large pot over medium heat. Add onion, garlic, mushrooms, carrot, and celery. Sauté for 5 minutes until vegetables start to soften.

Add pearl barley, vegetable broth, dried thyme, salt, and pepper. Bring to a boil.

Reduce heat and simmer for 40-45 minutes until barley is tender.

Adjust seasoning if needed. Serve hot.

Split Pea Soup:

What You Need

1 tablespoon olive oil

1 onion, chopped

2 cloves garlic, minced

2 cups dried split peas

6 cups vegetable broth

1 carrot, diced

1 celery stalk, diced

1 teaspoon dried thyme

Salt and pepper to taste

Directions

Heat olive oil in a large pot over medium heat. Add onion and garlic. Sauté for 5 minutes until onion is translucent.

Add dried split peas, vegetable broth, carrot, celery, dried thyme, salt, and pepper. Bring to a boil.

Reduce heat and simmer for 1 hour until split peas are tender.

Use an immersion blender or transfer a portion of the soup to a blender and blend until desired consistency.

Adjust seasoning if needed. Serve hot.

Butternut Squash Soup:

What You Need

1 tablespoon olive oil

1 onion, chopped

2 cloves garlic, minced

1 butternut squash, peeled, seeded, and cubed

4 cups vegetable broth

1 teaspoon dried sage

1/2 teaspoon nutmeg

Salt and pepper to taste

Directions

Heat olive oil in a large pot over medium heat. Add onion and garlic. Sauté for 5 minutes until onion is translucent.

Add butternut squash, vegetable broth, dried sage, nutmeg, salt, and pepper. Bring to a boil.

Reduce heat and simmer for 20-25 minutes until butternut squash is tender.

Use an immersion blender or transfer a portion of the soup to a blender and blend until smooth.

Adjust seasoning if needed. Serve hot.

Cabbage Soup:

What You Need

1 tablespoon olive oil

1 onion, chopped

2 cloves garlic, minced

4 cups vegetable broth

1 small head cabbage, shredded

2 carrots, diced

2 celery stalks, diced

1 can diced tomatoes

1 teaspoon dried thyme

Salt and pepper to taste

Directions

Heat olive oil in a large pot over medium heat. Add onion and garlic. Sauté for 5 minutes until onion is translucent.

Add vegetable broth, shredded cabbage, carrots, celery, diced tomatoes (with juice), dried thyme, salt, and pepper. Bring to a boil.

Reduce heat and simmer for 20 minutes until vegetables are tender.

Adjust seasoning if needed. Serve hot.

Turkey Chili:

What You Need

1 tablespoon olive oil

1 onion, chopped

2 cloves garlic, minced

1 pound ground turkey

1 bell pepper, diced

1 can diced tomatoes

1 can kidney beans, drained and rinsed

2 tablespoons chili powder

1 teaspoon cumin

Salt and pepper to taste

Directions

Heat olive oil in a large pot over medium heat. Add onion and garlic. Sauté for 5 minutes until onion is translucent.

Add ground turkey and cook until browned.

Add bell pepper, diced tomatoes (with juice), kidney beans, chili powder, cumin, salt, and pepper. Stir well.

Bring to a boil, then reduce heat and simmer for 20 minutes.

Adjust seasoning if needed. Serve hot.

Cauliflower Soup:

What You Need

1 tablespoon olive oil

1 onion, chopped

2 cloves garlic, minced

1 head cauliflower, chopped

4 cups vegetable broth

1 cup low-fat milk

1 teaspoon dried thyme

Salt and pepper to taste

Directions

Heat olive oil in a large pot over medium heat. Add onion and garlic. Sauté for 5 minutes until onion is translucent.

Add cauliflower and vegetable broth. Bring to a boil.

Reduce heat and simmer for 20 minutes until cauliflower is tender.

Use an immersion blender or transfer a portion of the soup to a blender and blend until smooth.

Return soup to the pot. Add low-fat milk, dried thyme, salt, and pepper. Stir until heated through.

Adjust seasoning if needed. Serve hot.

Chicken Tortilla Soup:

What You Need

1 tablespoon olive oil

1 onion, chopped

2 cloves garlic, minced

2 boneless, skinless chicken breasts, cooked and shredded

1 can diced tomatoes

4 cups chicken broth

1 bell pepper, diced

1 jalapeño pepper, seeded and diced (optional)

1 teaspoon cumin

1 teaspoon chili powder

Salt and pepper to taste

Toppings: low-fat tortilla chips, shredded reduced-fat cheese, chopped fresh cilantro, lime wedges

Directions

Heat olive oil in a large pot over medium heat. Add onion and garlic. Sauté for 5 minutes until onion is translucent.

Add shredded chicken, diced tomatoes (with juice), chicken broth, bell pepper, jalapeño pepper (if using), cumin, chili powder, salt, and pepper. Stir well.

Bring to a boil, then reduce heat and simmer for 20 minutes.

Adjust seasoning if needed. Serve hot.

Serve the soup with low-fat tortilla chips, shredded reduced-fat cheese, chopped fresh cilantro, and lime wedges for toppings.

Gazpacho:

What You Need

4 large tomatoes, chopped

1 cucumber, peeled and chopped

1 red bell pepper, chopped

1/4 red onion, chopped

2 cloves garlic, minced

2 tablespoons olive oil

2 tablespoons red wine vinegar

1/2 teaspoon cumin

Salt and pepper to taste

Garnish: chopped fresh basil or parsley

Directions

In a blender or food processor, combine the tomatoes, cucumber, red bell pepper, red onion, garlic, olive oil, red wine vinegar, cumin, salt, and pepper.

Blend until smooth or desired consistency.

Adjust seasoning if needed.

Refrigerate for at least 1 hour to chill.

Serve cold and garnish with chopped fresh basil or parsley.

Sweet Potato and Black Bean Soup:

What You Need

1 tablespoon olive oil

1 onion, chopped

2 cloves garlic, minced

2 sweet potatoes, peeled and diced

4 cups vegetable broth

1 can black beans, drained and rinsed

1 teaspoon cumin

1/2 teaspoon smoked paprika

Salt and pepper to taste

Toppings: plain Greek yogurt, chopped fresh cilantro, lime wedges

Directions

Heat olive oil in a large pot over medium heat. Add onion and garlic. Sauté for 5 minutes until onion is translucent.

Add diced sweet potatoes, vegetable broth, black beans, cumin, smoked paprika, salt, and pepper. Stir well.

Bring to a boil, then reduce heat and simmer for 20 minutes until sweet potatoes are tender.

Adjust seasoning if needed.

Serve hot and top each serving with a dollop of plain Greek yogurt, chopped fresh cilantro, and a squeeze of lime juice.

Carrot Ginger Soup:

What You Need

1 tablespoon olive oil

1 onion, chopped

2 cloves garlic, minced

1 pound carrots, peeled and chopped

4 cups vegetable broth

1 tablespoon grated fresh ginger

1/2 teaspoon ground turmeric

Salt and pepper to taste

Directions

Heat olive oil in a large pot over medium heat. Add onion and garlic. Sauté for 5 minutes until onion is translucent.

Add chopped carrots, vegetable broth, grated ginger, ground turmeric, salt, and pepper. Stir well.

Bring to a boil, then reduce heat and simmer for 20 minutes until carrots are tender.

Use an immersion blender or transfer a portion of the soup to a blender and blend until smooth.

Adjust seasoning if needed. Serve hot.

Moroccan Chickpea Soup:

What You Need

1 tablespoon olive oil

1 onion, chopped

2 cloves garlic, minced

1 carrot, diced

1 celery stalk, diced

1 teaspoon ground cumin

1 teaspoon ground coriander

1/2 teaspoon ground cinnamon

1 can chickpeas, drained and rinsed

4 cups vegetable broth

1 can diced tomatoes

Salt and pepper to taste

Fresh cilantro for garnish

Directions

Heat olive oil in a large pot over medium heat. Add onion and garlic. Sauté for 5 minutes until onion is translucent.

Add diced carrot, diced celery, ground cumin, ground coriander, and ground cinnamon. Sauté for an additional 3 minutes.

Add chickpeas, vegetable broth, diced tomatoes (with juice), salt, and pepper. Bring to a boil.

Reduce heat and simmer for 15 minutes.

Adjust seasoning if needed. Serve hot, garnished with fresh cilantro.

Zucchini Soup:

What You Need

1 tablespoon olive oil

1 onion, chopped

2 cloves garlic, minced

3 zucchinis, chopped

4 cups vegetable broth

1 teaspoon dried basil

1/2 teaspoon dried thyme

Salt and pepper to taste

Directions

Heat olive oil in a large pot over medium heat. Add onion and garlic. Sauté for 5 minutes until onion is translucent.

Add chopped zucchinis, vegetable broth, dried basil, dried thyme, salt, and pepper. Stir well.

Bring to a boil, then reduce heat and simmer for 15 minutes until zucchinis are tender.

Use an immersion blender or transfer a portion of the soup to a blender and blend until desired consistency.

Adjust seasoning if needed. Serve hot.

Thai Coconut Curry Soup:

What You Need

1 tablespoon olive oil

1 onion, chopped

2 cloves garlic, minced

2 tablespoons Thai red curry paste

1 can coconut milk

4 cups vegetable broth

1 red bell pepper, thinly sliced

1 zucchini, diced

1 cup sliced mushrooms

1 cup snow peas

Juice of 1 lime

Salt and pepper to taste

Fresh cilantro for garnish

Directions

Heat olive oil in a large pot over medium heat. Add onion and garlic. Sauté for 5 minutes until onion is translucent.

Add Thai red curry paste and stir for 1 minute.

Add coconut milk, vegetable broth, red bell pepper, diced zucchini, sliced mushrooms, and snow peas. Bring to a boil.

Reduce heat and simmer for 15 minutes until vegetables are tender.

Stir in lime juice, salt, and pepper. Adjust seasoning if needed.

Serve hot, garnished with fresh cilantro.

Navy Bean Soup:

What You Need

1 tablespoon olive oil

1 onion, chopped

2 cloves garlic, minced

2 carrots, diced

2 celery stalks, diced

1 pound dried navy beans, soaked overnight and drained

6 cups vegetable broth

1 bay leaf

1 teaspoon dried thyme

Salt and pepper to taste

Directions

Heat olive oil in a large pot over medium heat. Add onion, garlic, carrots, and celery. Sauté for 5 minutes until vegetables start to soften.

Add soaked navy beans, vegetable broth, bay leaf, dried thyme, salt, and pepper. Bring to a boil.

Reduce heat, cover, and simmer for 1 to 1 1/2 hours until beans are tender.

Remove the bay leaf. Adjust seasoning if needed.

Serve hot.

DESSERT RECIPES FOR HYPERTHYROIDISM

Baked Apples with Cinnamon:

What You Need

2 apples

1 teaspoon cinnamon

1 tablespoon honey or maple syrup

Optional toppings: chopped nuts, raisins, or a dollop of Greek yogurt

Directions

Preheat the oven to 375°F (190°C).

Wash the apples and remove the cores.

Place the apples in a baking dish.

In a small bowl, mix together the cinnamon and honey/maple syrup.

Spoon the cinnamon mixture into the center of each apple.

Optional: Sprinkle the optional toppings over the apples.

Bake for about 25-30 minutes or until the apples are soft and tender.

Remove from the oven and let them cool slightly.

Serve warm.

Greek Yogurt Parfait with Berries:

What You Need

1 cup Greek yogurt

1 cup mixed berries (such as strawberries, blueberries, raspberries)

2 tablespoons granola or crushed nuts

Optional: drizzle of honey or maple syrup

Directions

In a glass or bowl, start with a layer of Greek yogurt.

Add a layer of mixed berries on top of the yogurt.

Sprinkle a tablespoon of granola or crushed nuts over the berries.

Repeat the layers until all the What You Need are used.

Optional: Drizzle a small amount of honey or maple syrup on top.

Serve immediately.

Chia Pudding with Almond Milk:

What You Need

1/4 cup chia seeds

1 cup unsweetened almond milk (or any other non-dairy milk)

1-2 tablespoons honey or maple syrup

Optional toppings: fresh fruits, nuts, or shredded coconut

Directions

In a bowl, combine the chia seeds, almond milk, and honey/maple syrup.

Stir well to ensure the chia seeds are evenly distributed.

Let the mixture sit for about 5 minutes, then stir again to prevent clumping.

Cover the bowl and refrigerate for at least 2 hours or overnight.

Once the chia seeds have absorbed the liquid and formed a pudding-like consistency, give it a final stir.

Serve the chia pudding in individual bowls or glasses.

Add your desired toppings, such as fresh fruits, nuts, or shredded coconut.

Enjoy chilled.

Chocolate Avocado Mousse:

What You Need

2 ripe avocados

1/4 cup cocoa powder

1/4 cup honey or maple syrup

1/4 cup almond milk (or any other non-dairy milk)

1 teaspoon vanilla extract

Directions

Cut the avocados in half, remove the pits, and scoop out the flesh into a blender or food processor.

Add the cocoa powder, honey/maple syrup, almond milk, and vanilla extract.

Blend until smooth and creamy, scraping down the sides as needed.

Taste and adjust the sweetness if desired.

Transfer the mousse to serving bowls or glasses.

Refrigerate for at least 1 hour to allow it to set.

Serve chilled.

Coconut Flour Pancakes with Berries:

What You Need

1/4 cup coconut flour

1/4 teaspoon baking powder

Pinch of salt

2 eggs

1/4 cup almond milk (or any other non-dairy milk)

1 tablespoon honey or maple syrup

1/2 teaspoon vanilla extract

Fresh berries for topping

Directions

In a bowl, whisk together the coconut flour, baking powder, and salt.

In a separate bowl, beat the eggs.

Add the almond milk, honey/maple syrup, and vanilla extract to the beaten eggs. Mix well.

Pour the wet What You Need into the dry What You Need and stir until well combined.

Let the batter sit for a few minutes to allow the coconut flour to absorb the liquid.

Heat a non-stick skillet or griddle over medium heat.

Spoon about 2 tablespoons of batter onto the skillet for each pancake.

Cook until bubbles form on the surface, then flip and cook the other side until golden brown.

Repeat with the remaining batter.

Serve the pancakes with fresh berries on top.

Steamed Pears with Honey and Walnuts:

What You Need

2 ripe pears

2 tablespoons honey

2 tablespoons chopped walnuts

Directions

Peel the pears and cut them into halves, removing the cores.

Place the pear halves in a steamer basket or a heatproof dish.

Drizzle the honey over the pears and sprinkle with chopped walnuts.

Steam the pears over medium heat for about 10-15 minutes, or until they are tender.

Remove from the steamer and let them cool slightly.

Serve warm.

Pumpkin Spice Energy Balls:

What You Need

1 cup rolled oats

1/2 cup pumpkin puree

1/4 cup almond butter

1/4 cup honey or maple syrup

1 teaspoon pumpkin pie spice

1/4 cup unsweetened shredded coconut (for rolling, optional)

Directions

In a bowl, combine the rolled oats, pumpkin puree, almond butter, honey/maple syrup, and pumpkin pie spice.

Stir until all the What You Need are well combined.

Place the mixture in the refrigerator for 15-30 minutes to firm up.

Once chilled, roll the mixture into small bite-sized balls.

Optional: Roll the energy balls in shredded coconut for an additional coating.

Store the energy balls in an airtight container in the refrigerator until ready to serve.

Enjoy as a quick and energizing snack.

Almond Butter Banana Bites:

What You Need

2 ripe bananas

2 tablespoons almond butter

Optional toppings: crushed nuts, shredded coconut, dark chocolate chips

Directions

Peel the bananas and cut them into thick slices.

Spread a small amount of almond butter on half of the banana slices.

Top with another banana slice to create a "sandwich."

Optional: Roll the edges of the banana bites in crushed nuts, shredded coconut, or dark chocolate chips for added flavor and texture.

Place the banana bites on a tray lined with parchment paper.

Freeze for at least 1 hour until firm.

Serve the almond butter banana bites chilled.

Berry Sorbet (using natural sweeteners):

What You Need

2 cups mixed berries (such as strawberries, blueberries, raspberries)

1 tablespoon honey or maple syrup

1 tablespoon lemon juice

Directions

In a blender or food processor, combine the mixed berries, honey/maple syrup, and lemon juice.

Blend until smooth and well combined.

Taste the mixture and adjust the sweetness if desired.

Pour the mixture into a shallow dish or a loaf pan.

Cover with plastic wrap and place in the freezer for about 4-6 hours, or until the sorbet is firm.

Remove from the freezer and let it sit at room temperature for a few minutes to soften.

Scoop the sorbet into bowls or cones.

Serve immediately.

Quinoa Pudding with Mixed Berries:

What You Need

1/2 cup cooked quinoa

1 cup almond milk (or any other non-dairy milk)

2 tablespoons honey or maple syrup

1/2 teaspoon vanilla extract

Mixed berries for topping

Directions

In a saucepan, combine the cooked quinoa, almond milk, honey/maple syrup, and vanilla extract.

Stir well and bring the mixture to a gentle simmer over medium heat.

Cook for about 10-15 minutes, stirring occasionally, until the pudding thickens.

Remove from heat and let it cool slightly.

Transfer the quinoa pudding to serving bowls or glasses.

Top with mixed berries.

Serve warm or chilled.

Baked Peaches with Greek Yogurt Topping:

What You Need

2 ripe peaches

1 tablespoon honey or maple syrup

1/4 teaspoon cinnamon

1/4 cup Greek yogurt

Optional toppings: chopped nuts, granola

Directions

Preheat the oven to 375°F (190°C).

Cut the peaches in half and remove the pits.

Place the peach halves in a baking dish, cut side up.

Drizzle honey or maple syrup over the peaches.

Sprinkle cinnamon evenly over the peaches.

Bake for about 15-20 minutes or until the peaches are soft and slightly caramelized.

Remove from the oven and let them cool slightly.

In a small bowl, mix the Greek yogurt until smooth.

Serve the baked peaches with a dollop of Greek yogurt on top.

Optional: Sprinkle with chopped nuts or granola for added crunch.

Raw Vegan Chocolate Truffles:

What You Need

1 cup dates, pitted

1/2 cup raw cacao powder

1/2 cup almond meal

2 tablespoons coconut oil

Optional toppings: shredded coconut, chopped nuts, cacao powder

Directions

Place the dates in a food processor and process until they form a sticky paste.

Add the cacao powder, almond meal, and coconut oil to the processor.

Process until all the What You Need are well combined and a sticky dough forms.

Scoop out small portions of the dough and roll them into balls using your hands.

Optional: Roll the truffles in shredded coconut, chopped nuts, or cacao powder for different coatings.

Place the truffles on a plate or tray lined with parchment paper.

Refrigerate for at least 30 minutes to allow them to firm up.

Serve the raw vegan chocolate truffles chilled.

Grilled Pineapple Slices with Cinnamon:

What You Need

1 pineapple, peeled and cored

1 teaspoon cinnamon

Optional: a drizzle of honey or maple syrup

Directions

Preheat the grill to medium-high heat.

Slice the pineapple into rings or wedges.

In a small bowl, mix the cinnamon with a pinch of honey or maple syrup (optional).

Brush the pineapple slices with the cinnamon mixture on both sides.

Place the pineapple slices on the grill and cook for 2-3 minutes per side until grill marks appear and the pineapple is heated through.

Remove from the grill and let them cool slightly.

Serve the grilled pineapple slices as is or with a drizzle of honey or maple syrup if desired.

Dark Chocolate-Dipped Strawberries:

What You Need

1 cup dark chocolate chips or chopped dark chocolate

1 pint fresh strawberries, washed and dried

Directions

Line a baking sheet with parchment paper.

In a microwave-safe bowl, melt the dark chocolate chips or chopped dark chocolate in 30-second intervals, stirring in between, until fully melted and smooth.

Hold a strawberry by the stem and dip it into the melted chocolate, swirling to coat it completely.

Lift the strawberry out of the chocolate and let the excess chocolate drip off.

Place the chocolate-dipped strawberry on the prepared baking sheet.

Repeat the process with the remaining strawberries.

Once all the strawberries are dipped, place the baking sheet in the refrigerator for about 15-20 minutes to allow the chocolate to harden.

Remove from the refrigerator and serve.

Lemon Poppy Seed Muffins (using whole grains):

What You Need

1 cup whole wheat flour

1/2 cup almond flour

1/4 cup coconut sugar or honey

1 tablespoon poppy seeds

1 teaspoon baking powder

1/4 teaspoon baking soda

Pinch of salt

1/2 cup unsweetened almond milk (or any other non-dairy milk)

1/4 cup coconut oil, melted

Zest and juice of 1 lemon

1 teaspoon vanilla extract

Directions

Preheat the oven to 350°F (175°C).

In a large bowl, whisk together the whole wheat flour, almond flour, coconut sugar/honey, poppy seeds, baking powder, baking soda, and salt.

In a separate bowl, whisk together the almond milk, melted coconut oil, lemon zest, lemon juice, and vanilla extract.

Pour the wet What You Need into the dry What You Need and stir until just combined. Do not overmix.

Divide the batter evenly into a muffin tin lined with paper liners.

Bake for 15-18 minutes or until a toothpick inserted into the center of a muffin comes out clean.

Remove from the oven and let the muffins cool in the tin for a few minutes before transferring them to a wire rack to cool completely.

Serve the lemon poppy seed muffins at room temperature.

SECTION 5: LAST NOTE

As we come to the end of our exploration into managing hyperthyroidism through diet, we sincerely hope that this cookbook has provided you with fresh insights, valuable knowledge, and a renewed sense of empowerment over your health journey. Dealing with hyperthyroidism requires a comprehensive approach that encompasses professional medical care, thoughtful attention to nutrition and lifestyle choices, and a deep understanding of your own body.

It's crucial to recognize that managing hyperthyroidism is a highly individualized experience. What works best for one person may not necessarily be the ideal solution for another, and that's perfectly okay. Each individual's journey with hyperthyroidism is unique, and it's essential to embrace this diversity while navigating your path to wellness. By fostering open communication with your healthcare team, staying attuned to your body's signals, and integrating insights gained from research and discussions, you can take proactive steps towards optimizing your health and well-being.

This cookbook has been crafted to equip you with a diverse array of resources, including recipes, concepts, and considerations, to support you on your journey. Our greatest wish for you is to feel empowered to make informed decisions that enhance your quality of life, whether it involves fine-tuning nutrient balance, adapting dietary restrictions, or managing symptoms effectively.

Remember, you are not alone on this journey. Drawing upon the support of your loved ones, engaging in candid conversations with your healthcare provider, and maintaining an open-minded approach can all contribute to improving your thyroid health and overall well-being. Never underestimate the power you hold to shape your own health destiny, and recognize that your commitment to self-care is truly commendable.

May this cookbook serve as a steadfast companion and a wellspring of wisdom as you navigate life's twists and turns. We wish you resilience, self-compassion, and unwavering dedication to your health as you continue to manage your hyperthyroidism. May you find joy in a lifetime of good health and fulfillment.